THE ANXIETY BOOK

OF INSPIRATIONAL

QUOTES FOR THOSE

DIFFICULT DAYS.

"What upsets people is not things themselves but their judgements about these things."

Epictetus

"The only thing we have to fear is fear itself."

Franklin D. Roosevelt

"Worry often gives a small thing a big shadow."

Swedish Proverb

"The greatest mistake you can make in life is to be continually fearing you will make one."

Elbert Hubbard

"That the birds of worry and care fly over your head, this you cannot change, but that they build nests in your hair, this you can prevent."

Chinese Proverb

"Don't let yesterday take up too much of today."

Will Rogers

"When everything seems to be going against you, remember that the airplane takes off against the wind, not with it."

Henry Ford

"The journey of a thousand miles begins with a single step."

Lao Tzu

"One day you will tell your story of how you've overcome what you're going through, and it will become part of someone else's survival guide."

Unknown

"Reading is to the mind, what exercise is to the body."

Joseph Addison

"To keep the body in good health is a duty...otherwise, we shall not be able to keep our mind strong and clear."

Buddha

> *"Sometimes people with the worst past create the best future."*

Umar ibn al Khatab

"Life is a balance of holding on and letting go."

Rumi

"Happiness is the only good. The time to be happy is now. The place to be happy is here. The way to be happy is to make others so."

Robert Ingersoll

"If you want to be happy, be."

Leo Tolstoy

> *"I will either find a way or make one."*
>
> *Hannibal*

"The beginning is perhaps more difficult than anything else, but keep heart, it will turn out all right."

Vincent Van Gogh

"A crust eaten in peace is better than a banquet partaken in anxiety."

Aesop

"There is only one way to happiness and that is to cease worrying about things which are beyond the power of our will."

Epictetus

"My life has been full of terrible misfortunes - most of which have never happened."

Michel de Montaigne

"People become attached to their burdens sometimes more than the burdens are attached to them."

George Bernard Shaw

"When the winds of change blow, some people build walls and others build windmills."

Chinese Proverb

"Those who mind don't matter and those who matter don't mind."

Unknown

"What you think, you become. What you feel, you attract. What you imagine, you create."

Buddha

"Life is like riding a bicycle. To keep your balance, you must keep moving."

Albert Einstein

"Don't let your pizza go cold because you are busy looking at someone else's toppings."

Unknown

"Throw off your worries when you throw off your clothes at night."

Napoleon Bonaparte

"For every minute you are angry, you lose 60 seconds of happiness."

Ralph Waldo Emerson

"We can complain because rose bushes have thorns, or rejoice because thorn bushes have roses."

Abraham Lincoln

"The darkest hours are just before the dawn."

English Proverb

"Action may not always bring happiness; but there is no happiness without action."

Benjamin Disraeli

"You can never cross the ocean until you have the courage to lose sight of the shore."

Christopher Columbus

"If you fell down yesterday, stand up today."

H. G. Wells

"*Good humor is a tonic for mind and body. It is the best antidote for anxiety and depression.*"

Grenville Kleiser

"Today I escaped anxiety. Or no, I discarded it, because it was within me, in my own perceptions — not outside."

Marcus Aurelius

"If you want to lift yourself up, lift up someone else."

Booker T. Washington

"Nothing in life is to be feared. It is only to be understood."

Marie Curie

"We are more often frightened than hurt; and we suffer more from imagination than from reality."

Seneca

"Happiness depends upon ourselves."

Aristotle

"Tension is who you think you should be. Relaxation is who you are."

Chinese Proverb

"Never stop being a good person because of bad people."

Unknown

"Whenever you feel bad, just remember that Coca-Cola only sold 25 bottles in its first year. Never give up."

Unknown

"You can't change how people treat you or what they say about you. All you can do is change how you react to it."

Mahatma Gandhi

"Our greatest enemies, the ones we must fight most often, are within."

Thomas Paine

"This too shall pass."

Persian Proverb

"A little bit of light pushes away a lot of darkness."

Jewish Proverb

"Happiness grows at our own firesides and is not to be picked in stranger's gardens."

Douglas Jerrold

"Stand up to your obstacles and do something about them. You will find that they haven't half the strength you think they have."

Norman Vincent Peale

"The key is to keep company only with people who uplift you, whose presence calls forth your best."

Epictetus

"*Every tomorrow has two handles. We can take hold of it with the handle of anxiety or the handle of faith.*"

Henry Ward Beecher

"Fall Down seven times, get up 8."

Japanese Proverb

"If a person doesn't know to which port they sail, no wind is favourable."

Seneca

"We consume our tomorrows fretting about our yesterdays."

Persius

"No garden is without its weeds."

Thomas Fuller

"A man who fears suffering is already suffering from what he fears."

Michel de Montaigne

"*Do not worry about what others are doing! Each of us should turn the searchlight inward and purify his or her own heart as much as possible.*"

Mahatma Gandhi

"The best time to plant a tree was 20 years ago. The second best time is now."

Chinese Proverb

"Until you spread your wings, you'll have no idea how far you can fly."

Napoleon Bonaparte

"We build too many walls and not enough bridges."

Isaac Newton

"It is better to change an opinion than to persist in a wrong one."

Socrates

"Your teacher can open the door, but you must enter by yourself."

Chinese Proverb

"Anxiety weighs down the heart, but a kind word cheers it up."

Proverbs 12:25

"Most folks are about as happy as they make their minds up to be."

Abraham Lincoln

"Peace comes from within. Do not seek it without."

Buddha

"When you arise in the morning, think of what a precious privilege it is to be alive – to breathe, to think, to enjoy, to love."

Marcus Aurelius

"What is, is.
Accept."

Malcolm Inayat Omar

"Remember the time you thought you never could survive? You did and you can do it again."

Unknown

"Failure is not falling down but refusing to get up."

Chinese Proverb

"What is the point of dragging up sufferings that are over, of being miserable now, because you were miserable then?"

Seneca

"You yourself as much as anybody in the entire universe deserve your love and affection."

Buddha

"Don't judge each day by the harvest you reap but by the seeds that you plant."

Robert Louis Stevenson

"Man is not worried by real problems so much as by his imagined anxieties about real problems."

Epictetus

"God grant me the serenity to accept the things I cannot change, courage to change the things I can, and the wisdom to know the difference."

Reinhold Niebuhr

"There is a time to take counsel of your fears, and there is a time to never listen to any fear."

George S. Patton

"Fear: False Evidence Appearing Real."

Unknown

"The person who removes a mountain begins by carrying away small stones."

Chinese Proverb

"Most people don't realise the strength it takes to pull yourself out of a panic attack. So, if you have ever done that, be proud of yourself."

Unknown

"Care about what other people think and you will always be their prisoner."

Lao Tzu

"Anxiety isn't something you should ever apologise for."

Unknown

> *"He has the most who is most content with the least."*

Diogenes

*"**Anxiety does not empty tomorrow of its sorrows, but only empties today of its strength.**"*

Charles Spurgeon

"The secret of getting ahead is getting started."

Mark Twain

"It is better to be alone than in bad company."

George Washington

"Always concentrate on how far you've come, rather than how far you have left to go."

Unknown

"Believe you can and you are halfway there."

Theodore Roosevelt

"True happiness is to enjoy the present, without anxious dependence upon the future, not to amuse ourselves with either hopes or fears but to rest satisfied with what we have, which is sufficient, for he that is so wants nothing."

Seneca

"If we had not winter, the spring would not be so pleasant; if we did not sometimes taste of adversity, prosperity would not be so welcome."

Anne Bradstreet

"If you want happiness for an hour, take a nap. If you want happiness for a day, go fishing. If you want happiness for a year, inherit a fortune. If you want happiness for a lifetime, help someone else."

Chinese Proverb

"Apprehension, uncertainty, waiting, expectation, fear of surprise, do a patient more harm than any exertion."

Florence Nightingale

"The secret of happiness is to count your blessings while others are adding up their troubles."

William Penn

"**When one door closes, another opens; but we often look so long and so regretfully upon the closed door that we do not see the one which has opened for us.**"

Alexander Graham Bell

"Happiness is as a butterfly which, when pursued, is always beyond our grasp, but which if you will sit down quietly, may alight upon you."

Nathaniel Hawthorne

"Difficult roads often lead to beautiful situations."

Unknown

"You have power over your mind -- not outside events. Realise this and you will find strength."

Marcus Aurelius

"What is to give light must endure burning."

Viktor Frankl

"Nothing is permanent in this wicked world, not even our troubles."

Charlie Chaplin

"Always bear in mind that your own resolution to succeed is more important than any other."

Abraham Lincoln

"Sometimes the best therapy is listening to great music."

Unknown

"Dream of the life you want to live. Then live your dream."

Unknown

Printed in Great Britain
by Amazon

74455492R00061